VEGETARIAN KETO DIET FOR BEGINNERS

Lose Weight, Boost Brain Power, and Increase Your Energy

KAREN COLE

Contents

Introduction v
1. Ketogenic Diet 1
2. Plant-Based Diets 13
3. The New Keto 23
4. Ketotarian Foods 32
5. Practical Ketotarian and How to Get Started 40
6. Intermittent Fasting and Other Tips 45
7. The Recipes and Meal Plans 53
8. Ketotarian and Diabetes 69
9. Ketotarian and The Environment 73

Conclusion 79

© Copyright 2019 by Karen Cole - All rights reserved.

The following book is reproduced below with the goal of providing information that is as accurate and reliable as possible. Regardless, purchasing this book can be seen as consent to the fact that both the publisher and the author of this book are in no way experts on the topics discussed within and that any recommendations or suggestions that are made herein are for entertainment purposes only. Professionals should be consulted as needed prior to undertaking any of the action endorsed herein.

This declaration is deemed fair and valid by both the American Bar Association and the Committee of Publishers Association and is legally binding throughout the United States.

Furthermore, the transmission, duplication, or reproduction of any of the following work including specific information will be considered an illegal act irrespective of if it is done electronically or in print. This extends to creating a secondary or tertiary copy of the work or a recorded copy and is only allowed with the express written consent from the Publisher. All additional right reserved.

The information in the following pages is broadly considered a truthful and accurate account of facts and as such, any inattention, use, or misuse of the information in question by the reader will render any resulting actions solely under their purview. There are no scenarios in which the publisher or the original author of this work can be in any fashion deemed liable for any hardship or damages that may befall them after undertaking information described herein.

Additionally, the information in the following pages is intended only for informational purposes and should thus be thought of as universal. As befitting its nature, it is presented without assurance regarding its prolonged validity or interim quality. Trademarks that are mentioned are done without written consent and can in no way be considered an endorsement from the trademark holder.

Introduction

Congratulations on purchasing *Vegetarian Keto Diet for Beginners* and thank you for doing so.

The fact that you have downloaded this book means you are probably curious about how the vegetarian and ketogenic diets intersect. Both diets have become very popular in recent years. The ketogenic diet has been producing astonishing weight loss results while the health benefits of plant-based diets have been lauded by many doctors and physicians. There has also been a recent shift towards supporting more sustainable agriculture which has led many people to begin reducing their meat consumption. It is only natural then, that people have started to merge these two diets together.

The following chapters will discuss the key concepts of the

ketogenic and plant-based diets. We will look at where these diets intersect and the resulting benefits of the new keto diet or ketotarian diet as it's now being referred to. We will look at the specific nutritional benefits of different foods and provide you with recipes and meal plans to suit your lifestyle and dietary preferences as well as giving you practical information, we also dive deeper into broader topics such as the relationship between the ketotarian diet and the environment.

There are plenty of books on this subject on the market, so thanks again for choosing this one! I hope that it gives you a comprehensive understanding of everything you wanted to know about the diet and practical ways to incorporate this way of living into your everyday life. I hope you enjoy it!

Ketogenic Diet

What is the keto diet?

The ketogenic diet has become very popular recently. Its weight loss results have encouraged millions of people to start following this diet. People have also seen improvements in their overall health, which makes many people see it as a sustainable diet in the long term.

The basic concept behind the keto diet focuses on a majority intake of high-quality fat, a lower intake of protein and minimal carbohydrate intake. The breakdown tends to be roughly 75% fat, 20% protein, and just 5% carbohydrates. The purpose of the low carbohydrate intake is to lead the body into a state of ketosis.

What is ketosis?

Ketosis occurs when there is not enough glucose in the body. Glucose is normally used by the body to produce energy. Therefore, when glucose levels are too low, the body must look elsewhere for energy. This results in the body burning fat stores instead. The burning of fat stores results in a buildup of acids in the body. These acids are referred to as ketones. The ketone molecules are then used as the main source of energy for the body.

There is a transitionary period for the body as it switches fuel sources from glucose to ketones and sometimes this can result in a phenomenon called the "keto flu". As the body is not used to being in a regular state of ketosis, it may produce symptoms such as reduced energy and nausea for the first few days.

The Problem with Regular Diets

In most regular diets, ketosis rarely occurs. That is because most diets consist of high intakes of carbohydrates. When someone eats carbohydrates, the stomach breaks the food down into glucose, which is basically sugar for the body. This is the quickest form of energy the body can produce. This energy can either be used instantly by the body or else it is stored in the bloodstream for later use. The problem occurs when too much glucose is stored in the bloodstream. This causes blood sugar levels to become high. This is dangerous for people who are diabetic or at risk of diabetes. Next, the pancreas secretes insulin through the bloodstream which is used to help transport the glucose throughout the body. The act of eating carbohydrates triggers insulin to be secreted. The role of the insulin is to counteract the rising glucose levels occurring in the body. It does this by entering the bloodstream and transporting glucose to other parts of the body. This is why an overload of carbohydrates is risky for a diabetic patient as they cannot produce enough insulin to counteract the rising blood sugar levels.

Why and How Keto Works

By increasing the amount of fat and restricting the number of carbohydrates an individual consumes, the body is forced to switch to an alternate source of energy. Unable to create glucose due to a lack of carbohydrates, it now uses the excess fat stores for energy. During this process (ketosis), the fatty acids in your liver are converted into ketones. Ketones provide a more sustained dose of energy than glucose due to the fact that this is being created from high-quality fats. The body then burns up these ketones for energy. Because these ketones come from excess fat stores in the body, it enables the body to burn more fat than a regular high-carb diet.

What are the main foods in the Keto diet?

Now we will take a quick look at the main foods recommended to someone on a keto diet. In chapter 4, we will discuss the specific nutritional qualities some of these foods contain and the benefits of each nutrient on the body and mind.

Here are some of the most popular foods eaten on keto:

- Seafood: Oysters, mussels, clams, and squid
- Non-starchy vegetables: Broccoli, cauliflower, zucchini, cabbage, spinach
- All cheese
- Avocado
- Meat and poultry
- Eggs
- Coconut oil
- Plain Greek Yogurt
- Olive oil
- Seeds and nuts
- Berries
- Cream and butter
- Cocoa powder and dark chocolate

Benefits of the keto diet

Now we will look at a comprehensive list of the proposed benefits of adopting a keto lifestyle. There have been many studies undertaken over the past few years to try and solidify some of these findings. As always, there are counter-arguments to some of these benefits which we will cover in the next section.

Aids in weight loss

As mentioned previously, the process of ketosis, which burns excess fat stores in the body, aids significantly in weight loss for individuals. What happens during ketosis is that the blood sugar and insulin levels drop. This allows for the fat cells to release any water they have been retaining. This results in a large initial weight loss in individuals which is mostly due to this loss of water.

Over time, however, usually after a period of two to four days of keto dieting (although it can take a few weeks in some cases), the body begins switching fuel source from glucose to the amount of carbohydrates you are consuming, your body will be in a regular caloric deficit, contributing to continued weight loss during the period of your diet.

Another benefit of keto is that it helps control appetite. Most keto foods are high-fat and help you feel full. This results in less unhealthy food cravings and further aids in weight loss.

Improved mental focus

One of the problems with a carbohydrate-based diet is that energy in the form of glucose causes blood sugar levels to rise and fall intermittently. This leads to energy highs and lows which makes it difficult for your brain to remain focused over long periods of time.

In contrast, fueling your body using fat as the main fuel source results in having a more consistent source of fuel to rely on. This allows for longer periods of sustained focus.

When ketones are produced, they improve the efficiency of

the mitochondria. Mitochondria converts oxygen and nutrients into chemical energy. This energy is used by the cells of the body and the brain to help it function.

Increased Energy

Many people on the keto diet report having more physical energy throughout the day. Yet again this goes back to switching fuel source from glucose to fat. Your body has plenty of fat stores available to draw energy from when needed. As a result of this constant fuel injection, people have reported having higher levels of sustained energy.

Increases levels of HDL cholesterol

Firstly, cholesterol isn't all bad. It is an essential fat needed by cells in the body. Some of our cholesterol comes from the food we eat, and the rest is made in our liver. Cholesterol is unable to dissolve in the blood, so it must be carried throughout the body using proteins. We call these lipoproteins.

Keto has shown to increase levels of HDL cholesterol. HDL stands for high-density lipoprotein. These are also known as "good" cholesterol. HDL carries cholesterol towards the liver. Here, it is either excreted or re-used in the body. HDL cholesterol is thought to help reduce the risk of heart disease and stroke.

LDL, on the other hand, is referred to as "bad" cholesterol. LDL stands for low-density lipoprotein. LDL is a tiny blob of cholesterol with an outer rim of lipoprotein. LDL can build up with plaque, which can lead to clogged arteries. This can cause heart attacks and strokes.

Hence, having a high HDL cholesterol level is good and people should make sure to keep their levels of LDL cholesterol low. Keeping the LDL cholesterol low can be attained if food intake is also calculated and the type of food included in the diet is well-planned.

Helps prevent and reduce symptoms of diabetes

As the keto diet focuses on forcing the body to use fat for energy instead of glucose, it helps significantly decrease blood sugar levels and thus prevent insulin surges. This is great for people suffering from diabetes as regular occurrences of high blood sugar levels has many negative health consequences. These can include loss of vision and poor blood circulation, sometimes resulting in loss of limbs. The keto diet is also beneficial for those with pre-diabetic symptoms or those at risk of diabetes as they avoid reaching that dangerous state where blood sugar levels become high too frequently.

Reducing epileptic seizures in children

Numerous studies have linked the keto diet to help reduce the number of epileptic seizures in children, and in some cases, it has been deemed to help cure it.

The ketogenic diet is recommended by numerous health

organizations as a treatment for children with epilepsy, especially for those with seizures that are not controlled by AEDs (Anti-Epileptic Drugs). AEDs help prevent seizures by lowering the electrical activity of neurons in the brain. Excessive activity is what usually causes seizures.

They suggest that the keto diet can help lower the number of seizures a child experiences. It can also reduce the severity of these seizures. It has even been linked to leading to improved behavior.

Most people with epilepsy can control their seizures using anti-epileptic drugs. For those children who continue to have seizures despite the use of the drug, the ketogenic diet could be tried as a helpful alternative.

Reducing dementia and Alzheimer's disease

Some studies have also found that older adults, who were at higher risk of decreased brain function, experienced better functioning memory after only six weeks on the keto diet.

As mentioned, ketones have shown to increase the efficiency of mitochondria, giving more energy to the brain. As well as this, ketones have also shown to improve synapses signals between neurons, reduce inflammation in the brain and lower oxidative stress.

Alzheimer's disease causes the brain to no longer accept glucose as a fuel source as the brain becomes resistant to insulin. This helps explain why the rates of Alzheimer's disease are higher among diabetics.

This has led many to suggest using the keto diet to help divert the effects of Alzheimer's disease. While the logic for the argument of using ketones is solid, it is still seen as an untested approach by most researchers and doctors in the field. There has only been a small number of clinical trials performed on humans that tests the theory.

The few clinical studies that were undertaken so far suggested that the diet helped those with mild Alzheimer's better than any of the current medicines. Despite these findings, many more clinical trials need to be performed in order to validate the diet's effects. However, there are no current risks to the diet so it's probably worth a shot for those suffering from the condition.

Helps fight cancer

The keto diet has also been linked with fighting cancer. In general, cancer therapies aim at targeting cancer cells, which are biologically different to normal cells. Most cancer cells feed off carbohydrates (glucose) which enables them to multiply.

As we've seen, the glucose levels in the blood go down during a keto diet. This is presumed to be good in the fight against cancer as it helps starve the cancer cells, preventing them from growing in number.

Like any other living organism, cancer cells also need food to survive. Over a period of time, the keto diet can theoretically not only prevent the cancer cells from growing in number, but they can also cause them to decrease in size and possibly even die.

Therefore, it does seem possible that a ketogenic diet could help in a person's fight against cancer due to its ability to significantly reduce blood sugar levels.

Criticisms of the Keto Diet

No diet is without its critics and it's worth mentioning some of the counter-arguments to the benefits of the keto diet. In order to gain a full understanding of any diet, it is important to look at all sides of the discussion to enable you to make your own informed decision on what you think is best for you.

1. *A prolonged state of ketosis is unhealthy*

Some critics suggest that putting the body in a constant state of ketosis is neither healthy nor natural. Ketosis makes the blood more acidic and it is a mild form of ketoacidosis which is a very dangerous state where the blood becomes overly acidic. However, ketoacidosis is usually only experienced by those with type one diabetes and not through a keto diet.

1. *Keto is not specifically responsible for reducing the effects of*

seizure

Some critics also suggest that, while there is a clear *correlation* between children adopting the keto diet and a reduction in epileptic seizures, the diet itself is not the *cause* for that reduction. They argue that the reduction is due to children moving away from their old diets of highly processed foods, such as children's breakfast cereals and processed meats.

Processed food is defined by any food that is altered by a number of mechanical or chemical operations intended to either change it or preserve it. They typically come packed in a box or bag and contain more than one ingredient. Not all processed foods are necessarily bad. Some foods which are only mechanically processed can still be healthy. Take apple sauce for example. If the apples are cored, peeled and then cooked to make apple sauce they are still healthy. These are mechanical processes. However, if refined sugar and artificial flavors were then added to the sauce to enhance the taste, then it would also become chemically processed. It is these chemically processed foods that all of us should try to avoid, if possible. Over-consumption of these processed foods leads to a series of health problems.

Thus, some people argue that any diet which eliminates the dependence on highly-processed foods will garner the same results as the keto diet.

1. *Keto is not responsible for reducing the effects of cancer*

A recent study has found that highly-processed foods are strongly linked with increasing the risk of cancer. Highly-processed foods are those with additives such as salt, sugar, artificial flavors/colors, preservatives, and emulsifiers.

The study entitled *'Consumption of ultra-processed foods and cancer risk'* took place in France and studied over 100,000 individuals. The study found that a 10% increase in the amount of ultra-processed foods in a person's diet was linked with a higher than 10% increase in their risk of cancer. The study cannot determine with certainty however, that the increased cancer risk is directly caused by these ultra-processed foods. In theory, it could also be due to a lack of nutrients from healthy foods that the other not-at-risk participants were getting more benefit from.

The same criticism is also held for the suggestion that the keto diet helps improve memory function. Critics insist that the same results would be seen with any low-carb diet where there are less processed foods consumed.

1. *Overconsumption of cholesterol is bad for you*

Despite the arguments from the keto community about the importance of defining good cholesterol versus bad cholesterol, some people believe that over-consuming cholesterol in your diet and increasing the cholesterol levels in the body will result in putting a person at risk of heart disease.

2

Plant-Based Diets

What is a plant-based diet?

Another type of diet that is very popular today is a plant-based diet. People have been choosing plant-based diets for a multitude of reasons. Some of the main ones include:

- being concerned about how animals are being treated
- believing plant-based diets are better for overall health
- coming under social pressure from friends and family to move away from meat
- being concerned about the impact of agriculture on the environment

Before we move further, however, I want to inform you that there are many variations of plant-based diets. There can be large variances between these diets, especially when looking at the standard vegan diet versus the standard vegetarian diet. I'm going to give you a general overview of all the different plant-based diets, but I will focus mainly on vegan and vegetarian diets for the rest of the chapter.

Plant-based diets are, yes, you guessed it, mainly focused on plant-based foods. However, most plant-based diets also put a large focus on whole foods. This refers to natural foods that are not heavily processed. The main foods eaten in plant-based diets tend to be fruits, vegetables, legumes, whole grains, nuts, and seeds. There also tends to be very few or no animal products.

What is a vegan?

The basic definition of a vegan is someone who doesn't eat or use any animal products. This includes meat, fish, dairy, eggs, and honey. Vegans refrain from using or promoting the use of clothes, shoes, shampoos or any other product that has been made using animal material. In most cases, being a vegan is more than just a diet, it is a lifestyle choice. Most vegans aim to lead by example in the fight against animal cruelty and they often aim to shed a light on the many social, environmental and ethical problems occurring in the agriculture industry today.

What is a vegetarian?

The definition of a vegetarian is someone who abstains from eating meat. Therefore, unlike vegans, vegetarians may still eat cheese, eggs, and other types dairy products. They may also still use animal products such as leather or fur for clothing or other items.

Given the broad definition of a vegetarian, people have begun to group into different subsections of vegetarians based on what foods they eat.

- A *Lacto ovo vegetarian* is a person who eats eggs and other dairy products. They are the most basic form of vegetarian, only refusing to eat meat.
- A *lacto vegetarian* is a person who also does not eat eggs. They may consume other dairy products however, such as milk, butter or cheese.
- An *ovo-vegetarian* is a person who eats eggs but doesn't eat dairy.
- A *pescatarian* is a person who eats fish and shellfish.
- *Semi-vegetarians* (or *flexitarians*) occasionally eat meat or poultry.

What's the difference between plant-based, vegan and vegetarian?

Plant-based vs Vegan: Vegans hold a philosophy that is devoted to protecting animals from unnecessary cruelty. Being a vegan is more than just a diet, it is a lifestyle that promotes equality for all sentient beings. Vegans remove animal products from every aspect of their lives, including their diet. This means using no clothes or accessories made of fur, wool or leather. It also means not consuming products such as honey which have originated from insects or using any shampoos or make-up that may have been tested on animals.

Plant-based diets, on the other hand, refer to the whole, plant foods. These include fruits, vegetables, nuts, seeds, legumes, and whole grains. This is more specific than just allowing all vegan foods. For example, Oreo cookies and fries are technically vegan, but they are not plant-based. This is because neither product is in their original plant form. While plant-based meals are technically all vegan, someone following a plant-based diet may still not be a vegan. They may still wear and consume clothes and other accessories that use animal products.

Vegan vs Vegetarian: When comparing a typical vegan diet to a typical vegetarian diet, more focused use of dairy products in the vegetarian diet is the core difference between the two. While the vegetarian diet only restricts people eating meat, the vegan diet restricts the consumption or use of any animal products. This means being a vegan requires much more awareness about ensuring you know exactly what ingredients are in the foods you are consuming. Certain food items which most would presume are vegan-friendly might not be. For example, there are certain brands of peanuts that contain an animal-based gelatin to make them taste saltier. In cases like this, a vegan should try to make sure to buy organic peanuts.

What are the main foods on a plant-based diet?

Here we will list the most popular foods eaten on a plant-based diet. Keeping in mind the many variations of plant-based diets that exist, we will focus on the general plant-based philosophy and not that of other plant-based diets. This means our list will not include pescatarian acceptable foods (fish and shellfish) and vegetarian acceptable foods (eggs and dairy).

Here are some of the most popular foods eaten on a plant-based diet:

- Non-starchy vegetables: Broccoli, spinach, zucchini, cabbage, tomatoes
- Starchy vegetables: Potatoes, yams, chickpeas, beans, peas, corn, lentils
- Fruits: Apples, bananas, citrus, strawberries, grapes
- Whole grains: oats, whole wheat, brown rice
- Drinks: water, unsweetened coffee, and tea, unsweetened plant kinds of milk
- Omega 3s: Flax seed, chia seeds
- Spices: All spices

Benefits of plant-based diets

There has been a large push towards plant-based diets in recent years due to the large number of health benefits associated with eating a whole food, plant-based diet. Some of the main benefits include:

Help keep our heart healthy

Many plant-based foods including legumes, nuts, seeds, whole grains, and fruits tend to have high levels of potassium. Potassium aids in lowering blood pressure. It is very important to prevent blood pressure levels from getting too high for risk of heart problems. Potassium is also great for relieving anxiety and stress. Most meats contain little or no potassium and thus these benefits aren't found on high-cholesterol diets.

Plants also contain no cholesterol compared with the high levels of cholesterol in eggs and meat. Even saturated plant sources such as coconut contain no cholesterol. Although keto-dieters will like to argue that it is important to consider bad and good cholesterol levels, plant-based dieters believe that consuming high cholesterol foods such as eggs and meat is linked with an increased risk of heart disease. They believe that by eating plant-based foods you will eliminate the chance of your cholesterol levels going too high.

Help prevent type 2 diabetes

Part of the reason a plant-based diet helps prevent diabetes is that most people on plant-based diets tend to control their weight better than those eating diets high in meat and carbohydrates. Carrying too much body fat is the main cause of someone acquiring type 2 diabetes. Roughly 90% of people who develop type 2 diabetes are overweight. People on a plant-based diet tend to have lower obesity levels than those on other regular diets.

Another reason for the reduction in type 2 diabetes and sometimes the elimination of the disease is that there are very little saturated fats in plant-based products. Saturated fats that are found in high quantities in meat and dairy result in insulin resistance. This is the exact cause of type 2 diabetes. The fats in plant-based foods are mostly monounsaturated. These are found in foods such as olive oil, avocados, and certain nuts. These fats protect against the adverse effects of saturated fats.

Therefore, people who eat plant-based foods tend to have safer blood sugar levels and greater insulin sensitivity. This is important for allowing blood sugar to enter the cells in your body.

Help prevent arthritis

Osteoarthritis is the most common cause of disability in older people. It is a joint disease resulting from the breaking down of joint cartilage. The main cause for the breakdown of this cartilage is shown to be inflammation. Inflammatory foods include meat and dairy as well as refined grains and sugar. Too much consumption of these food places the immune system in an oxidative state and causes low-grade systemic inflammation.

It is also shown that levels of rheumatoid arthritis are greater in countries where meat and dairy are consumed in larger quantities. This is also an inflammatory disease which causes long-term pain and swelling in the joints. By avoiding meat and dairy products, plant-based eaters are less susceptible to these diseases.

Help prevent cancer

Plant-based diets have been shown to reduce the risk of cancer. Even for those who have already been diagnosed with cancer, it has been seen to help them through it and sometimes recover from it.

Meat and dairy foods have both been linked to certain cancers. Red meat and processed meat often contain carcinogens, which have the potential to cause cancer. Consumption of dairy has also been suggested as contributing to certain cancers such as prostate cancer and ovarian cancer.

Many experts suggest a colorful, plant-based diet in helping you stay healthy in the fight against cancer. More color in your diet means a more diverse mix of nutrients that can have cancer-fighting properties. Beta-carotene is what gives sweet potatoes its unique color and the same for lycopene in tomatoes. Both compounds help your body against cancer.

Also, fiber is found in abundance in plant-based foods. Fiber helps in the removal of excess hormones in the body which can cause certain cancers

Criticisms of plant-based diets

Plant-based diets lack sufficient protein

When switching to a plant-based diet, making sure to consume enough protein is very important. When moving from a diet of high-protein meats, it is easy for someone to not consciously concern themselves with their amount of protein intake. Many people who support naturally high-protein diets, such as those high in quantities of meat and dairy, suggest that these animal products are necessary for your body to get all the protein it needs to function. While it is possible to get protein from plant-based sources such as brown rice, beans, and nuts, critics believe most plant-based eaters do not consume enough.

Plant-based diets lack sufficient calcium

Another argument against plant-based diets is that they lack enough amounts of calcium. Many supporters of diets high in animal products suggest it is important to consume meat and dairy to get enough levels of calcium. Calcium is available in plant-based foods such as kale, spinach, and almonds but critics say these sources are not plentiful enough.

Plant-based diets lack vitamin B12

Probably the biggest concern for those on a plant-based diet is the inability to get enough vitamin B12 in their diet. The only plant-based foods containing B12 are those that have been fortified with B12 such as certain plant milk and soy products. However, the quantities supplied in these foods tend not to be enough for most people's needs. That is why it is recommended that people on a plant-based diet use supplements such as fish oils to raise their vitamin B12 levels. The only real source of the B12 vitamin is in fish, meat, eggs, or dairy. Thus, meat-eaters argue that because there is no naturally occurring B12 vitamin in plants, it suggests eating meat and dairy products should be natural and is important for our health.

3

The New Keto

What is the New Keto?

The ketotarian diet is a new diet which was recently created by Dr. Will Cole. It follows the basic rules of the standard ketogenic diet, but it looks at it from a plant-based perspective. This means it also has a high emphasis on consuming healthier fats, a moderate amount of protein and a few carbs. To be clear, however, this diet is not a vegetarian version of keto. Dr. Cole still sees a place in his diet for healthy meats on occasion. Grass-fed beef, as well as pasture-raised pork, are some of the healthy and sustainable meat options that Dr. Cole suggests can be eaten once or twice a week. The first eight weeks of the diet should be focused solely on plant-based foods but after this period, some kinds of meats can be introduced. While meat, fish, and eggs are still accepted on the ketotarian diet, they are meant to be eaten in moderation. This differentiates it from the standard keto diet where high levels of these foods are consumed. Alternatively, the majority of ketotarian foods are plant-based foods containing healthy fats. This includes foods such as avocados and nuts as well as vegetables such as dark leafy greens.

The philosophy behind it

Dr. Will Cole had been a strict vegan for ten years. As a student in college, he had educated himself on things such as factory farming and concentrated animal feeding operations. He discovered the terrible conditions the animals we eat are forced to live in. He also discovered the effects that eating these animals has on our health and the devastating effects it has on pollution and the environment. Armed with this knowledge he made the decision to become a vegan.

Once Will started studying functional medicine, however, things began to change. He realized the importance of getting to the root cause of an illness. He also realized that the same treatment doesn't work for everyone. While he was eating a diet that he knew was healthy, he was feeling unhealthy. At this point, he knew something was wrong and that he must change something.

So, after ten years of being a vegan, he decided to quit. He began the search for a new diet that would enable him to live a healthier life. Although veganism was surely better than the standard American diet, it wasn't the optimal choice for Will.

Problems experienced on a vegan diet

Issues with digestion

Will believes that abstaining from healthy, organic meats had an impact on his digestion. By running functional medicine labs on himself, he discovered that he had developed hypochlorhydria and gallbladder issues. Hypochlorhydria is where the production of acid in gastric secretions of the stomach is low. Both issues made it hard for his body to digest food. He was also eating large portions of grains and legumes. Together, this contributed to him developing the leaky gut syndrome.

Weak detox pathways

Will, along with around 40% of the population has methylation problems. Methylation is a biochemical process that involves transferring an active methyl group across different molecules. It is required for everything from DNA synthesis to detoxification. It also helps greatly with our immune health.

In order to have healthy methylation pathways, we need to have enough vitamins B9 and B12 as well as choline. Wild fish is the best natural source for finding all these nutrients. These nutrients could also be supplemented but Will believes it is better to get them naturally and thus, wild fish is part of the ketotarian diet.

Unhealthy skin

Will's skin had always been prone to acne. Through his vegan diet, he was unable to get enough good vitamin A. This, combined with his poor gut health, led to him having unhealthy skin.

Plant carotenes can be found in carrots and sweet potatoes. Through the metabolic process, these can be converted to vitamin A. The problem is that the rate of conversion to usable retinol is poor. Retinol is what's often referred to as true vitamin A. It is vitamin A in its bioavailable form. Retinol is only present in certain animal products. The main sources include fish, eggs, and cod liver oil.

Once Will started incorporating cod liver oil into his diet, he noticed a remarked improvement in his skin health.

Weak immune system

While on a strict vegan diet Will often found himself feeling run down. While he was missing out on consuming enough healthy fats, he was also not getting enough fat-soluble vitamins. In order to have a strong immune system, you need sufficient quantities of vitamin A. Not having enough vitamin A can cause autoimmune diseases like type 1 diabetes and rheumatoid arthritis.

Vitamin D has also been proven to be key in maintaining

the body's metabolism and immune health. It is also found abundantly in fish, eggs, and ghee (a grass-fed Indian-style butter). The sun is also a great source of vitamin D. It is recommended to try and get between 20 and 60 minutes of sunshine a day in order to improve your levels of vitamin D. You can usually tell when someone isn't getting enough vitamin D as they tend to look more pale than usual.

Another important vitamin that is not as well-known, is K2. Most people on Western diets don't receive enough of this vitamin in their diets. Ghee also contains vitamin K (as well as vitamins A and D) which makes it an excellent food for getting all three of these nutrients. Another source of vitamin K is natto. This is a food which originated in Japan and it is made using non-GMO fermented soybeans.

Problems experienced on a ketogenic diet

While Will was experiencing problems with his strict vegan diet, he also realized there were lots of problems people were also having on a strict ketogenic diet. The below are a sample of some of the issues that arose when people turned to keto diets.

Loss in muscle

Some studies have shown that muscle loss can happen to people while on a ketogenic diet. This could possibly be related to the fact protein also needs carbs to aid in the building of muscle. Losing muscle can have serious consequences as we get older and it is important to ensure that we track changes in muscle mass with dietary changes.

Stress on Kidneys

One of the potential side effects of the keto diet is developing kidney stones. This has been seen in studies of children using the keto diet to treat their epilepsy. Roughly 7% of participants developed kidney stones. The likelihood of getting kidney stones fell when children consumed potassium citrate.

What experts believe leads to kidney stones on a keto diet is a high intake of processed meats as well as too much animal proteins which can cause high amounts of uric acid.

Bowel problems

The keto diet tends to neglect a lot of foods which are rich in fiber. The amount of whole grains, fruit and beans tend to be restricted which leads to a lack of enough fiber in the body. Fiber is necessary for normal laxation and it is good for the microbiome. The importance of the microbiome is huge to our immune health. As a result, many people suffer from constipation while on a keto diet.

Benefits of the ketotarian diet

The ketotarian diet takes a more holistic view of the keto and plant-based diets, pulling the top benefits from both and merging them into one complete and healthy diet. The less restrictive nature of the ketotarian diet also opens a way for vegans, vegetarians and pescatarians to join in the benefits of keto too.

Below are some of the benefits you can hope to find on the ketotarian diet:

Utilizing the power of ketosis

One of the fundamental principles behind the ketotarian diet is harnessing the power of ketosis. The general rule of the ketogenic diet is still followed on the ketotarian diet, with 75% of foods consumed being healthy fats, 20% being protein and roughly 5% carbs. This allows ketotarians to still reap the benefits of the traditional keto diet such as weight loss, lower levels of inflammation, improved brain health and improved energy.

Lower blood sugar

We have seen that significantly limiting our intake of carbohydrates helps reduce the levels of glucose in the blood, thus, lowering our blood sugar levels. Due to the same limitations on carbohydrates in ketotarian diet as seen in regular keto diet, the benefits here are the same. Thus, lower blood sugar helps minimize the risk of diabetes and can even cure type 2 diabetes over time.

Improve detox pathways

Will's detox problems, along with those experienced by many plant-based eaters, were solved with the introduction of wild caught fish into the diet. Wild fish is the best source of vitamins B9, B12, and choline which are all important in helping detox the body.

Improve immune system

Allowing for a few portions of fish each week helps prevent the problem many vegans have in being unable to get vital nutrients such as vitamin A, vitamin D. Ghee, and natto which are included in the diet also provide the necessary amount of vitamin K2 which many plant-based eaters also lack. Getting enough of these nutrients helps keep the immune system healthy.

Helps prevent heart disease

We have seen that one of the benefits of both the keto diet and the plant-based diet are their ability to help prevent heart disease.

Helps prevent cancer

Both keto and plant-based diets have shown results to help fight off cancer.

The main reason for this is the elimination of carbohydrates and high-processed foods. In keto, it is said that cancer cells need glucose to grow and multiply. Thus, limiting sugar in the diet helps starve these cancer cells.

In the plant-based diet, however, it is suggested that consuming meat also has strong links to producing cancer.

This is true for certain red meats and processed meats which produce carcinogens when cooked.

The key difference in the ketotarian diet, however, is that meat consumption is limited to once or twice per week, thus, keeping levels of possible carcinogens low. Processed meats are also not recommended on the ketotarian diet but rather organic, grass-fed meats which do not contain the same unhealthy hormones found in processed meat.

As mentioned previously, beta-carotene found in sweet potatoes, lycopene in tomatoes and fiber found in most vegetables also help the body against cancer.

Improved kidney function

Restricting the consumption of processed meats and only allowing for occasional grass-fed meats helps reduce the negative effects that eating processed meat has on the kidneys.

4

Ketotarian Foods

In this chapter, we are going to look at the main food groups that make up the ketotarian diet. We will look at exactly what foods you should be choosing from each group and the nutrients they contain.

Seafood

Fish and shellfish are excellent sources of food for people on the ketotarian diet. Most fish are very low in carbohydrates yet high in vitamin B, selenium, and potassium. However, some shellfish do contain a higher amount of carbs which needs to be noted. While this is not necessarily a reason to exclude them from your diet, it is important to make sure you are aware of which ones they are if you are trying to keep within a specific carb range.

Below we have included the carb counts of some popular

types of shellfish for your reference: The number of grams (denoted by g) is based on 100g servings:

- Mussel - 7g
- Clam - 5g
- Squid - 3g
- Oyster - 4g

High-fat fish such as salmon, mackerel, and sardines contain high rates of omega-3. Omega-3 is an anti-inflammatory acid which has shown to have very positive health benefits. It helps prevent heart disease and has also been shown to improve mental disorders such as depression and schizophrenia.

Having said this, it is important not to get carried away with the benefits of omega-3. Taking overly excessive quantities of polyunsaturated fatty acids comes with a series of health risks. Omega-3 and omega-6 are two such polyunsaturated fats that we find in our diets. They can lead to the production of free radicals. These tend to cause cell damage which perpetuates aging and can sometimes lead to cancer.

High amounts of omega-6 are found in processed seed and vegetable oils. Corn, sunflower, cottonseed, and soybean oil have high omega-6 amounts and should be avoided if possible. Choose alternatives such as butter, lard, coconut oil, and olive oil instead. The reason to avoid oils high in omega-6 is that having a high intake of omega-6 fatty acids compared with omega-3 may promote chronic disease. Since the industrial era, people have been consuming much higher levels of omega-6 than our pre-industrial ancestors. Our omega-6 to omega-3 ratio now sits around 16:1 where it previously reached highs of only 4:1. People living in Inuit communities, who mostly ate fish that was rich in omega-3, had ratios as low as 1:4. This means most people are already living with high ratios of omega-6 in their bodies. While eating more omega 3 can help counteract this ratio, it is more important to try and maintain a relatively low, balanced amount of omega-3 and omega-6.

Based on the research, having at least two servings of seafood in a week helps give you a good balance of omega-3 fats. Sticking to oils and other cooking fats low in omega-6 will also help keep the omega ratio healthy.

Meat

Meat is an optional choice in the ketotarian diet. When meat is added into the diet it is consumed very rarely, maybe only once or twice a week.

If meat is to be added it should always be organic, grass-fed meat. This type of meat contains very little carbs and is rich in vitamin B as well as minerals such as selenium, zinc, and potassium.

Meat is also a great source of protein, which can sometimes be lacking in vegetables.

Non-starchy vegetables

Non-starchy vegetables are excellent sources of nutrients, including vitamin C and multiple minerals. They are also very low in carbohydrates which is why they are strongly recommended on the ketotarian diet. The amount of carbohydrates in these types of vegetables vary between one and eight grams per cup.

Most vegetables have numerous antioxidants that enable the body to protect itself against free radicals. Free radicals are molecules that can inflict damage to the cells. They are very high in nutrients which helps lower the risk of disease.

Some of the most nutritional non-starchy vegetables include:

- **spinach:** vitamin A and K, protein, and fiber
- **broccoli:** vitamin C and K1, protein, and fiber
- **cabbage:** vitamin C, calcium, potassium, folic acid, and fiber
- **zucchini:** vitamin B1, potassium, manganese, and fiber
- **tomatoes:** vitamin C and beta-carotene
- **asparagus:** vitamin K1, protein, and fiber
- **kale:** vitamin A, C, and K1, protein and beta-carotene
- **carrots:** vitamins A and K, potassium and beta-carotene

- **green beans:** vitamin C, potassium and folic acid
- **leeks:** vitamins A and C, and fiber
- **peppers:** vitamins A, B6 and C, beta-carotene and potassium

Avocados

Avocados are one of the best foods for the ketotarian diet. They are extremely healthy and can be added to a variety of different meals. Due to their numerous health benefits, they are often referred to as a superfood.

In one full avocado (which is around 200 grams) there are 18 grams of carbs. However, 14 of the 18 grams accounts for fiber. So really the carb count is only 4 grams which is very low.

The avocado is full of healthy, monounsaturated fats. This is definitely perfect for the ketotarian diet.

Avocados contain nearly 20 vitamins and minerals including potassium. They are also salt-free, cholesterol-free and sugar-free. They also help increase the absorption of vitamins A, D, K, and E. In addition, avocados help further improve levels of cholesterol and triglyceride.

Coconut Oil

Coconut oil consists of medium-chain triglycerides. These are used by the liver to convert into ketones for energy. As a result of this, coconut oil is often used to treat people with Alzheimer's to help raise ketone levels.

Coconut oil contains medium chain fatty acids, referred to as MCFAs. These saturated fats help raise HDL ("good" cholesterol) which in turn lowers overall cholesterol levels and the risk of heart disease.

Coconut oil has also shown to increase metabolism leading to improved weight loss which is why it is imperative to include this in the ketotarian diet.

Olive Oil

Olive oil has a wide range of great heart benefits. It contains oleic acid which is a monounsaturated fat that helps lower the risk of heart disease. Extra-virgin olive oil is full of antioxidants which help reduce inflammation and protect the heart.

Olive oil contains zero carbohydrates and is excellent to use on salads or for cooking. However, it is best to use olive oil for low-heat cooking as it isn't as stable at high temperatures.

Nuts and Seeds

Nuts and seeds are an excellent and tasty addition to the ketotarian diet. They provide an easy snack and can be added to many types of dishes, including curries and salads.

Nuts and seeds are a great source of healthy fats and are

very high in protein and fiber. Consuming them regularly has shown to help reduce levels of cancer and heart disease.

While the majority of nuts and seeds have a low net carb count, they can vary among different types.

Below we have outlined the number of carbs per 28 grams of popular nuts and seeds:

- Almonds: 6g (3g fiber)
- Brazil nuts: 3g (2g fiber)
- Cashews: 9g (1g fiber)
- Macadamia nuts: 4g (2g fiber)
- Pecans: 4g (3g fiber)
- Pistachios: 8g (3g fiber)
- Walnuts: 4g (2g fiber)
- Chia seeds: 12g (11g fiber)
- Flaxseeds: 8g (8g fiber)
- Pumpkin seeds: 5g (1g fiber)
- Sesame seeds: 7g (4g fiber)

Berries

A small portion of fruits are recommended in the ketotarian diet and one of the most nutritious fruits available are berries.

Raspberries, blueberries, and blackberries are extremely high in antioxidants, the highest of any fruit. While the body needs a certain amount of free radicals to help fight bacteria and viruses, antioxidants help to keep your free radicals in check, before they become excessive and risk damaging your cells. Antioxidants also help prevent inflammation.

While berries may be higher in carbohydrates compared to other foods on the ketotarian diet, raspberries and blackberries also have high levels of fiber which lowers their net carb content. One cup of raspberries or blackberries has 15 grams of carbs, 8 of which is fiber.

Berries are very high in minerals and vitamins. One cup of strawberries produce 1.5 times your necessary intake of vitamin C for the day.

Looking at calories, berries have the lowest of any fruit. A cup of strawberries contains roughly 49 calories while a cup of blueberries has the highest of the berries at 84 calories.

5

Practical Ketotarian and How to Get Started

Step 1: What is your motivation?

Before you begin any new habit in life you should always ask yourself, "what is motivating me to do this?". If you do not have a strong and clear motivation for what you are doing, then you will fail. Once things start to get a little difficult you will fall at the first hurdle. You need to have a strong reason why you have decided to take on this diet. Maybe you suffer from a lack of energy all the time and you want to be at your best at work? Maybe there is a lot of heart problems in your family history and you don't want to follow the same fate? Maybe you are currently overweight and at risk of not seeing your children grow up if you don't do something about it? Whatever your personal motivation is, you must have it clear in your mind before starting. Write it down on a piece of paper and keep it with you in your wallet or purse. Or have it as the screensaver on your phone. Then when the tough times come, you will be able to remind yourself why you're doing what you're doing and that will give you the power to get through it.

Step 2: Decide what a ketotarian diet means for you

The next thing you need to do is decide how you want to structure your new diet. What foods do you want to include? Are you going to add some wild fish and grass-fed meat once or twice a week or are you going to solely focus on high-fat vegetables and stay completely plant-based? This diet is for you and you must first decide what foods you think you need most and what foods you think you will enjoy eating. While the diet specifically focuses on wholesome, high-fat, plant-based foods there is a lot of variety within that bracket. Food is one of the great pleasures in life and you need to look forward to your meals. If you don't enjoy the foods in your diet, then you are never going to stick with it. Make a note of what you want to include to make this diet be wholesome and enjoyable for you.

Step 3: Clean out the fridge and go shopping

Once you've decided what foods you are going to allow in your diet you must get rid of everything that didn't make the list. You may have tons of food in your home that is either processed or high in carbs and sugar. As difficult as it sounds you must grab some boxes and start packing them in. The only way to sustain the willpower to not go to the cupboard and grab a late-night snack of cookies is to have no cookies in the house. Willpower alone doesn't work in these situations, trust me! If you don't want to contribute to food waste, you can donate the food to the nearest food bank or homeless shelter. They will always be appreciative of having more food to hand out so you will be doing yourself and your community some good.

The next step is to go shopping for new foods you will be eating. Bring the list of your favorites and find a supermarket or a fruit and vegetables store nearby if possible - or else find one that is on your way to or from work. This will help make it easier for you to build a habit of shopping in the same place for the same foods at the same time each day (or every other day). The problem with a diet high in vegetables, such as the ketotarian diet, is that it requires regular shopping as most of the food is perishable after a few days.

Step 4: Talk with friends

It is difficult to build a new habit and one of the toughest barriers to building a successful one is getting enough support from your close friends and family. There are bound to be a few of them who don't agree with your new diet choices. But if they are your friends, hopefully, they will support your decision, regardless of whether they agree with the diet themselves. Once you make them aware that you are serious about making these changes, they will hopefully be more considerate of your dietary needs when going out for dinner together or when cooking at home in the case of your family.

Most people tend to be fairly accepting of people trying new diets these days but there tends to be always someone who feels the need to confront you on your choice. Instead of expanding unnecessary energy trying to justify your decision in an effort to convince these naysayers that you are right, simply don't bother. You don't need to justify yourself to anyone. If they do ask why just tell them you are doing it because you believe it will be good for you. I know this has made things much easier in my own life so give it a try!

Step 5: Pre-plan your meals

If you want to eat something healthy for lunch tomorrow that means you might need to purchase it today. Planning meals the night before helps us stick to our diet plans. Make sure to always bring some healthy snacks with you before you go somewhere. Fruit and nuts tend to be the easiest and best snacks to carry for the ketotarian diet. If you are going for a good few hours you may want to pack a proper lunch. Pre-planning what foods you are going to eat that day and bringing them with you significantly lowers the chances of you making impulse purchases of unhealthy snacks like chocolate bars in a store or croissants at a coffee shop.

Step 6: Have cheat days

While looking after your health and sticking to your new diet is important, it is also important to reward yourself now and again for your continued effort. There is no point living a longer and healthier life if you're completely miserable the whole time. One way to incorporate rewards into your diet is to have a cheat day once a week. This is a day where you can stray from your strict dietary routine. Where you can gorge on handfuls of sugar and carbs should you wish, and where you can decide to break your intermittent fasting schedule. Instead of staying at home to cook another vegetable-dense dinner, go out and buy a pizza!

Sticking to a strict diet can prove to be mentally tough over time. Having one day per week where you can relax and forget about the diet has shown to radically improve the chances of someone sticking to a diet. Without regular rewards, we will not stick to our habits and introducing cheat days is an important part of the habit building process.

Another benefit of a cheat day is that it prevents your metabolism from slowing down. Once your body gets used to consuming fewer calories, your metabolism can start to slow down over time. By having one cheat day per week, you are ensuring that it doesn't.

6

Intermittent Fasting and Other Tips

Intermittent Fasting

Intermittent fasting is a technique that is becoming increasingly popular due to its numerous health benefits. It involves fasting for long periods each day in order to give the digestive system a break. A lot of the body's energy is used on digesting food so by giving the digestive system a long break we are enabling the body's energy to be focused in other areas of repair and recovery. The optimum time to fast is for at least 15 hours out of a 24-hour day. This gives you a window of 9 hours in which you should consume all your necessary food.

Depending on your lifestyle and work schedule you will need to tweak the time periods in which you eat. For someone working in a typical 9 to 5 job, they may decide to not have their first meal until 11 am. This gives them until 8 pm that evening to have their last meal. This may sound difficult if you are somebody who is used to having breakfast in the morning but trust me, after a few days of trying it you won't even get hungry in the mornings.

Below are some of the benefits of intermittent fasting:

Increased weight loss

The main benefit seen from intermittent fasting is a better functioning metabolism. By eating the same quantity of food in a shorter time frame (9 hours or less) you can lose a significant amount of weight. Weight loss occurs because we are putting food into our bodies only while our metabolisms are most active. Our metabolisms work on a clock and once we eat our first piece of food or take our first sip of a drink in the morning that clock is set off. Any food or drink will set off the clock apart from water. The metabolism is at its best for the first 9 hours after it begins. Once it has been working over 9 hours it starts to slow down and it is at this point where people tend to put on more weight. As well as this, intermittent fasting helps release more of the fat burning hormone called norepinephrine.

Increased muscle growth

One of the benefits of intermittent fasting is increased muscle mass. Regardless of whether diet or exercise habits change, the rate of muscle growth can double during intermittent fasting. When we work out our muscles they break down. When we give the body more time and resources to repair itself, it rebuilds the muscles bigger and stronger.

Increased energy

Digesting food takes a lot of energy. By skipping breakfast and giving your digestive system a break, you will have increased energy in the mornings. Your body will be using the food that has been digested overnight to fuel you for the day.

Increased focus

Intermittent fasting can lead to more neurogenesis. Neurogenesis refers to the growth of new brain cells.

It has also shown to increase a protein in the brain called BDNF. This protein plays an important role in neuroplasticity, which is concerned with changes and adaptations of the brain that help make it less susceptible to stress. BDNF also aids in the production of brain cells and triggers new synapses and connections leading to improved memory, mood and learning capabilities.

Mindful Eating

Eating mindfully is a very important habit which is often overlooked today. Many people eat unconsciously and rush their meals, not being fully present in the experience. It is important to slow down and pause for a minute before you engage in eating your meal. You should also eliminate external distractions while you eat, such as watching tv, to give yourself the ability to focus fully on your food. There is a multitude of benefits to eating mindfully:

Puts the body and brain in sync

When we slow down our eating, we give the body time to send signals to the brain when we are starting to get full. The body takes around 20 minutes before it sends signals that it is full. Therefore, many of us overeat while rushing our food. We don't give the body enough time to catch up.

Connects us with our food

Eating more mindfully allows us to connect with our food better and enjoy the tastes and flavors more vividly. Developing a deep appreciation for the food on your plate and the nutrients it is giving has shown to increase the benefits you get from those nutrients.

Reminding you of your motivations

By focusing on enjoying each bite of your healthy meal, you are creating strong bonds between yourself and your commitment to a healthier lifestyle. You are reminding yourself about the journey you are on and why you choose these foods. By being more mindful and aware of what you are eating, you will be far less likely to unconsciously stray towards unhealthy options.

Drink lots of water

You should be drinking at least 2 liters of water each day to coincide with your new diet. Our bodies are made up of 60% water and there are a whole host of benefits to consuming water, especially first thing in the morning, which often go overlooked.

Helps you lose weight

Water naturally suppresses your appetite as it contains no cholesterol, calories or fat. It also helps to improve your metabolism.

Removes toxins

Water has the ability to naturally detoxify your body. It helps the body get rid of toxins through sweat and urination.

Improves your skin

Drinking plenty of water is excellent for your skin and acts as a natural moisturizer, keeping it soft and wrinkle-free.

Boosts immune system

Along with helping flush out harmful toxins from your body, water also helps carry oxygen to the body's cells.

Reduces headaches

Water helps reduce headaches by keeping your body from getting dehydrated. Dehydration causes the brain to slowly shrink from lack of fluid, which causes headaches.

Exercise

There has been plenty of science recently showing the benefits of regular exercise for both the brain and the body. A healthy diet mixed with a good exercise habit can significantly increase both the length and quality of your life.

While there are many different theories on the best type and optimum duration of exercise many studies have shown that either one hour of high-intensity exercise or ninety minutes of medium to high intensity per day is the sweet spot. Any more than that and you start getting diminishing returns from your workouts and sometimes even negative returns. Similar to the ketotarian diet, the key with exercise is getting the right balance for you. There are plenty of excellent and enjoyable exercises out there, from yoga to jogging to team sports. Choose one or two that you enjoy and that complement each other. For example, cycling and yoga. If you want to build an exercise habit, it's always better to choose something you enjoy doing (or if you don't enjoy it, at least something you feel better once it's finished!).

Some of the benefits of exercise:

Increases your happiness

Exercise reduces levels of stress in the brain and it also induces the release of hormones such as serotonin and norepinephrine which reduce feelings of depression. It also produces increased endorphins in the brain which help give you a positive feeling.

Aids in further weight loss

If you utilize the ketotarian diet, intermittent fasting, as well as some exercise, you are sure to be a weight loss machine!

Improves muscles and bones

Running, weight lifting and most other exercises help increase muscle growth. When doing activities that are strenuous on the muscles, make sure to up the intake of protein in your diet. Relatively high impact exercise also helps with increasing bone density and prevents bones from becoming weak over time.

Increases energy

Regular exercise doesn't drain your energy, it boosts it. Again, the important thing here is to not overdo the amount of exercise you have each day. Doing between 60 to 90 minutes of exercise in the mornings will leave you with a great injection of energy for the rest of your day.

Recover and Sleep

If exercise is one of the pillars to a healthy lifestyle, then sleep and recovery is another equally important pillar. One without the other will cause the building to collapse. Without proper recovery and sleep, all your hard work in exercising will just be in vain. In order to reap all the benefits of exercise, you must know how to recover properly.

In general, most people need between seven and nine hours of sleep every night. While there are some people out there who claim they get by on less than five, they are the exception to the rule. Our "always-on" working culture has tried to diminish the importance of sleep but the truth is it's vital to our overall health and energy levels. Suffering from a lack of sleep has the same effect on the brain as being intoxicated. We are unable to think clearly, our memory is foggy and our reactions are slowed. If you do need to get up at the crack of dawn, then go to bed earlier.

While we sleep, our brains and bodies are given a chance to recover from the day. Recovery in our brains means moving items from our short-term memory into our long-term memory. Recovery for our bodies means repairing muscles and tissues that have been broken down during exercise that day.

Along with sleep, another important part of the recovery process is consuming the right nutrients after exercise. Ensuring you get enough electrolytes after a run or enough protein after a weight session is the key to ensuring you get the maximum benefits from your exercise.

7

The Recipes and Meal Plans

Lunch Recipes

Veggie Greek Wraps

List of ingredients:

1 cup full-fat plain Greek yogurt

1 medium cucumber

1 Tbsp white vinegar

1 tsp garlic powder

½ block feta, cut into 4 (1-inch thick) strips

½ cup diced purple onion

½ medium red bell pepper

2 Tbsps. minced fresh dill

2 Tbsps. olive oil

70g seeded and grated cucumber

4 large halved cherry tomatoes

4 large collard green leaves

8 whole kalamata olives

Salt and pepper

How to make:

Mix the specified portions of Greek yogurt, garlic powder, white vinegar, olive oil, cucumber, fresh dill, salt, and pepper to together to make the tzatziki sauce.

Wash the leaves of the collard green wraps and trim the stem off each leaf.

Put two Tbsps. of tzatziki onto each wrap and spread

. . .

Add the cucumber, olives, feta, pepper, onion and tomatoes to the middle of the wrap.

Fold it over like a burrito.

Cut into halves and serve with any remaining tzatziki.

Mac and Cheese

List of ingredients:

1 ½ cups shredded cheddar cheese

1 medium cauliflower, riced

1 tsp turmeric

2 tsps. paprika

3 large eggs

¾ tsp rosemary

How to make:

Cut cauliflower into florets, making sure to get rid of stem.

Put the cauliflower in a food processor until it looks like rice.

Boil cauliflower for 4 mins.

Once cooked, wrap the cauliflower in a kitchen towel to get rid of excess water.

Put the cauliflower "rice" into a bowl.

Add eggs to the cauliflower. Add one egg at a time to ensure it doesn't become too watery.

Add cheddar cheese on top

Add your spices rosemary, turmeric, and paprika.

Mix everything together with your hands.

Heat olive and coconut oil in a pan on high heat.

Make the cauliflower mixture into a ball, and then flatten it.

. . .

Put these patty-style cauliflowers onto the pan and reduce heat to medium.

Flip until crisp on both sides.

Serve on a bed of spinach.

Stuffed Chickpea and Tuna Avocado

List of ingredients:

1/3 cup chickpeas

1/2 cup cilantro

1/2 cup quick pickled onions

1/2 tsp garlic powder

1/2 tsp pepper

1/2 tsp salt

1/2 tsp smoked paprika

1/4 cup feta

1/4 cup vegan chipotle sauce

2 large avocados

2 sliced radishes

2 tsp lemon juice

2 tsp olive oil

2 tsp za'atar

4 Tbsp Greek yogurt

5 oz tuna

How to make:

Add the 5 ounces of tuna along with the olive oil, za'atar, yogurt and lemon juice and stir together.

Put the chickpeas in a bowl, adding the smoked paprika, salt, pepper and garlic powder for seasoning.

Prepare avocados by cutting them in half and removing the stone. Fill up the avocados with the tuna mix and the now seasoned chickpeas.

Add radishes, cilantro, feta and the quick pickled onions. Finish it off by adding the vegan chipotle sauce.

Dinner Recipes

Cauliflower Steaks and Toasted Nuts with Romesco Sauce

List of ingredients:

1/8 tsp freshly ground black pepper

1/4 cup raw unsalted almonds, lightly toasted and chopped

1/4 cup roasted red bell peppers, drained

1/4 tsp ras el hanout seasoning

1/2 tsp sea salt

1 tsp minced fresh garlic

2 Tbsps. finely chopped fresh parsley leaves

2 Tbsps. sherry vinegar

3 Tbsps. olive oil

One 2 3/4-pound head cauliflower

How to make:

To begin you must preheat the grill to 350°F.

Cut the cauliflower in half down the middle, through the stalk. This will give you two large pieces of cauliflower (your steaks).

Remove any green from the cauliflower and make sure it is dry.

Mix together the ras el hanout with 2 Tbsps. oil, 1 Tbsp vinegar, and 1/4 tsp salt. Use about half of this mixture and brush it over the cauliflower

Put the cauliflower under the grill for 8 mins, until slightly blackened. Turn it over and cover with the rest of the oil mixture. Continue grilling for 10 more mins, or until cauliflower is nice and tender. Remove and cover with tinfoil.

Add the remaining 1 Tbsp vinegar, 1 Tbsp oil, 2 Tbsps. almonds, 1/4 tsp salt, garlic, bell peppers, and the black pepper to a food processor and grind until smooth.

Thinly slice the 2 Tbsps. almonds left. Cover the cauliflower with the remaining sauce and sprinkle with parsley and the sliced almonds.

Chili Tamari Tofu and Coconut Lime Noodles

List of ingredients:

1 block (400g) tofu

1 can (400ml) coconut milk

1 Tbsp olive oil

1/2 tsp ground or freshly grated ginger

1/4 tsp cayenne pepper (or ground chili pepper of choice)

1/4 tsp red pepper flakes

2 packages (8oz/226g each) shirataki noodles

4 tbsp low sodium tamari

4 tbsp sesame seeds

juice and zest of 1 lime

pinch of salt

How to make:

Heat the oven to 350F.

Drain out the tofu and cut it into roughly 1-inch by 1-inch blocks.

Mix the tamari, cayenne and olive oil. Layer the tofu cubes in a bowl. Pour the mix over the tofu. Turn the pieces of tofu to make sure they are completely covered.

Put the tofu on a baking tray and bake for 25 mins.

Meanwhile, drain the noodles. Place on a pan on medium heat, mixing in the rest of the noodle ingredients. Cook for 10 mins, then reduce heat and cook for 10 more mins.

Once finished, allow to cool and then garnish with lime zest, microgreens, red pepper flakes, and sesame seeds.

Sesame Tofu with Eggplant

List of ingredients:

1 cup fresh chopped cilantro

400g tofu

1 Tbsp olive oil

1 tsp crushed red pepper flakes

1 whole eggplant

¼ cup sesame seeds

¼ cup soy sauce

2 finely chopped cloves garlic

2 tsps. Swerve confectioners

3 Tbsps. unseasoned rice vinegar

4 Tbsps. toasted sesame oil

Salt and pepper

How to make:

Heat oven to 200°F. Drain the water from the tofu.

Put ¼ cup of cilantro, 3 Tbsps. rice vinegar, crushed red pepper flakes, minced garlic, 2 Tbsps. toasted sesame oil and Swerve into a mixing bowl and mix together.

Peel the eggplant and cut into strips. Mix the eggplant with your mixture.

Add the Tbsp of olive oil to a deep pan over medium heat. Cook the eggplant until it becomes soft.

Switch off the oven and add the leftover cilantro into the eggplant. Move the noodles into an oven dish and cover with a lid or tinfoil, leave in the oven to keep it warm.

Cut the tofu into 8 pieces. Put the sesame seeds onto a plate and press them into the tofu.

Put 2 Tbsps. of sesame oil onto the pan. Fry the tofu until they become crispy. Cover the tofu with ¼ cup of soy sauce while on the pan. Leave cooking until the tofu pieces look brown.

Remove the noodles from the oven and add the tofu.

Vegetable Tagine with Ghee Almonds and Olives (Moroccan style)

List of ingredients:

1/8 tsp ground cumin

1/8 tsp plus a dash of ground cinnamon

1/4 cup pitted green olives, halved

1/4 cup plus 1 Tbsp ghee

1/2 cup raw unsalted almonds, coarsely chopped

1 cup preservative-free, sugar-free vegetable broth or stock

1 small red onion, cut into small dice

1 small zucchini, cut into small dice

1 Tbsp tomato paste

1 tsp minced fresh garlic

1 tsp minced fresh ginger

1.5 cups packed fresh Swiss chard leaves, thinly sliced

2 Tbsps. finely chopped fresh cilantro or parsley leaves

2 yellow, orange, or red bell peppers, cut into small dice

3/8 tsp sea salt

Dash of cayenne pepper

How to make:

Put 2 Tbsps. of ghee in a deep pan over medium heat. Once hot, add garlic, ginger, bell peppers, onion, 1/8 tsp cinnamon, 1/4 tsp salt. Also add the cumin and cayenne and stir until onions are well done. Add in tomato paste and heat for 1 min.

Put in zucchini and cook until nice and soft. Add in chard and stir for another 3 mins. Add olives and broth and bring to boil. Cover pan and reduce heat to low. Simmer for 10 mins. Add in 2 Tbsps. of ghee and leave it to melt.

Heat the remaining 1 Tbsp of ghee in a separate pan over medium heat. Once it melts, add almonds, 1/8 tsp salt and a little bit of cinnamon. Cook almonds until light brown, careful to not let them burn.

Serve the tagine in bowls and top with cilantro and almonds.

Zucchini Ribbons

List of ingredients:

1 cup fresh basil leaves

1 Tbsp olive oil

½ cup water, if needed*

½ large avocado

½ large lemon

½ tsp salt

¼ cup Parmesan cheese, grated

¼ cup walnuts

2 cloves garlic, peeled

3 medium zucchini

5-6 leaves fresh basil, to garnish

Avocado Walnut Pesto

Salt and pepper

How to make:

Slice the zucchini into slim ribbons using a vegetable peeler, Stop peeling once you get to the seeds.

Put the ribbons in a colander and add salt.

Add the avocado, garlic, lemon, basil, walnuts, and cheese to a food processor and blend. Add water if necessary, to make the sauce nice and smooth.

Add 1 Tbsp olive oil to a pan and bring to medium heat.

. . .

Cook the zucchini ribbons roughly 5 mins until they start to become soft.

Add the pesto onto the zucchini ribbons.

Garnish with Parmesan cheese and fresh basil and serve.

Roasted Veg with Olive-Basil Pesto

List of ingredients:

1/4 cup plus 1 tsp olive oil

1/4 tsp coarse salt

1/2 cup pitted green olives

1 cup packed fresh basil leaves

1 to 2 tsps. finely ground spirulina

2 cups cremini mushrooms, halved

3 cups fresh Brussels sprouts, trimmed and halved

3 garlic cloves

3/4 cup thinly sliced red onion wedges

3/8 tsp freshly ground black pepper

How to make:

Turn on over to heat of 425°F. Put garlic onto a small sheet of tinfoil and pour 1 tsp oil over it. Completely wrap the garlic in the foil. Put in the oven and cook for 25 mins. The garlic should be tender and slightly brown.

Spread mushrooms, onion, Brussels sprouts, 2 Tbsps. oil, salt, and 1/4 tsp pepper in a large roasting pan. Put in the oven alongside the garlic, also for 25 mins Stir twice and cook until veg are tender and light brown.

Put the garlic cloves in a food processor along with olives. Blend together until nicely chopped. Add the leftover 1/8 tsp pepper as well as the basil and spirulina. Run processor again until the basil is nicely chopped. Add the leftover 2 Tbsps. oil. Run processor once more until the pesto is nearly smooth.

Split roasted vegetables onto two plates. Cover with pesto and serve.

8

Ketotarian and Diabetes

There is ongoing research about the effects the ketogenic diet and plant-based diets are having on both the rates of diabetes and the severity of its effects for both type 1 and type 2. While diet alone has been shown to cure type 2 diabetes, it is unknown as to whether it is possible to cure type 1. There are some key differences in both type 1 and type 2 diabetes so in this chapter we will look at them both separately.

Type 2 Diabetes

Type 2 diabetes is the most regular form of diabetes. Between 90 and 95 percent of people who have the disease have type 2 with the remaining 5 to 10 percent having type 1. Type 2 diabetes has become a health epidemic around the world with 422 million people suffering from the disease as of 2014 that is compared with only 108 million people having the disease in 1980. Type 2 diabetes is caused solely as a result of unhealthy living. Poor diets which are high in carbohydrates and refined sugars, as well as a lack of physical exercise, are the main factors resulting in people contracting the disease. The increasing amounts of processed foods on our store shelves and the relatively cheap costs of these foods is largely to blame for the significant increase in recent years.

As type 2 diabetes is caused as a result of unhealthy living, it can also be managed and even cured through healthy living. By losing weight, eating healthily and getting regular exercise while monitoring your blood sugar levels, people with the disease can continue to live as normal. In some more severe cases, people may need to add doses of insulin also.

However, it doesn't end there for people with type 2 diabetes. By committing to certain low-carb diets it has been shown that people can completely cure their type 2 diabetes.

How does the ketotarian help?

The ketotarian diet is the perfect diet for someone suffering from type 2 diabetes. By eliminating carbs, it helps to keep their blood sugar levels low and by focusing on healthy plant-based foods it gives them all the vitamins and minerals needed to keep their bodies optimally healthy for recovery from disease.

Type 1 Diabetes

Type 1 diabetes is a disease where the pancreas no longer produces insulin. Insulin is a hormone in the body that is necessary for controlling the level of glucose in the blood. Without insulin, the sugar in your blood builds up instead of being used as energy by the body. Your body makes its own sugar, but it also gets it from foods (mainly those high in carbs).

The causes of type 1 diabetes are still unclear. Current thinking on the subject believes that it happens as a result of the immune system mistakenly destroying the insulin-producing cells in the pancreas. Doctors believe there could possibly be other factors involved in the occurrence of the disease such as viruses and genetics.

How is it managed?

Type 1 diabetes takes a lot more management than type 2. Injections of insulin are required before every meal containing any amount carbs.

How does the ketotarian diet help?

Eating a healthy ketotarian diet can improve the fluctuations of blood sugar experienced by someone with type 1 diabetes. Constantly fluctuating blood sugar levels take a toll on the body and those with type 1 can suffer later in life as a result. Loss of vision and bad circulation in the feet leading to loss of limbs can be a scary result of not keeping blood sugar levels in check.

By eating a ketotarian diet, type 1 people may also be able to inject less insulin than usual as not all meals will contain carbs.

Is there a cure for type 1 diabetes?

While there is no cure for type 1 diabetes at present, there is a lot of ongoing research that suggests a cure is not far away.

Scientists in Denmark and Germany have discovered a potential future treatment in something called progenitor cells. These are regarded as earlier descendants of stem cells. The scientists have been able to determine where these progenitor cells in the pancreas are destined to become insulin-producing cells. If they can predetermine what are the necessary components for the development of an insulin-producing cell, then theoretically they should be able to recreate that cell structure in someone with type 1 diabetes.

9

Ketotarian and The Environment

There has been plenty of attention recently on the negative effects that the meat and dairy industry are having on the environment. We are going to look at some of the main environmental issues being caused by the current meat and dairy industry at present. We will also look at the effect switching to a ketotarian diet can have on these issues.

Climate change

The big problem on everyone's lips these days is global warming and climate change. There is no doubt that climates are changing but there has been a lot of debate on what the main causes are. For years, we believed the release of fossil fuels from factories and cars was the main culprit for destroying the ozone layer. Now, it is known that the effects of fossils fuels pale in comparison to the effect that the methane being released from cows is having on our environment. With the increasing number of cattle being bred for beef and milk production every year, the farming industry is causing devastating effects on the climate.

Food shortages

There is estimated to be enough food to feed the entire world more than twice over, yet millions still die from hunger each year. A lot of our surplus corn is being fed to cows instead of humans. While the amount of corn needed to feed one cow over its lifespan is speculative, one thing that is for sure is that if we stopped feeding this corn to cattle and used it in places where there are significant food shortages, hunger would be much less of an issue than it is today.

By moving away from corn-fed beef and putting more emphasis on grass-fed cattle, we can help to significantly reverse these food shortages. As well as this, the grass is much healthier for cows to consume as it is their natural food source. This provides us with healthier meat and dairy products as a result.

Clean-water shortages

The amount of water needed to produce beef is also causing serious water shortages. A 2013 study suggested that it takes 1,799 gallons of water to produce one pound of beef. While the accuracy of these numbers is often disputed by government and farming bodies, it is clear the beef industry has a lot to answer for in terms of its water usage.

The environmental impact of this water use could be devastating in the near future if supplies continue to decrease. It also poses ethical questions about whether this clean water should be used for more humanitarian causes.

Pollution

The amount of waste produced by cows and pigs is causing pollution of many rivers and lakes. This kills many of the wild fish and plankton. It also results in the spread of disease in areas where the water is used for drinking.

The poisoning of fish and plankton could have serious knock-on effects on the entire ecosystem. Plankton is the vital base to the oceanic food chain and without it, much of the fish in our seas and oceans will start to die out.

Soil erosion

The use of pesticides in growing crops has had devastating effects on the soil. Pesticides make their way down through the soil, killing all of the soil's nutrients. Once the soil loses its nutrients it becomes weak and over time, it is eroded away.

For profit-reasons, many of these huge farms harvest one single crop at a time to try and maximize yields. Not diversifying and rotating these crops regularly also kills the soil. Overgrazing the land with animals is another contributing factor to this problem.

Habitat loss

Huge amounts of forest land are being excavated each day to make way for new farm pastures. After destroying the soil in one area, farms move on to find fresh soil and repeat the unsustainable process of growing crops and killing all the soils nutrients. Forest land is home to a wide array of animals and once the trees are cut down, these animals become homeless. Many of them who are dependent on the forest habitat die as a result. The increasing level of deforestation for agriculture is putting many animal species at risk of extinction.

What can we do about it?

Besides lobbying your local politicians to introduce laws to implement improved and more sustainable farming methods, there are a few personal choices you can make to help the environment.

By choosing the ketotarian diet, you are already doing a better job than most as you are mainly focusing on whole foods and vegetables in your diet.

To really make an impact however, you should try and choose organic foods where you can afford it. Organic fruit and vegetables have been grown without the use of pesticides. While this is also much better for your health, it is also much better for the environment as it promotes a sustainable system of agriculture that doesn't destroy soil nutrients.

If you have decided to include meat and fish a few times a week you should choose organic, grass-fed beef, and wild-caught fish. Organic, grass-fed beef contains none of the unhealthy hormones that are present in regular meats and it promotes a more humane and sustainable way of farming. Choosing wild-caught fish also promotes sustainable fishing practice instead of buying from large fisheries. While the prices of these items may be slightly more, it shouldn't hurt your budget too much if you are only consuming them once or twice per week and it is well worth the health and environmental benefits.

Conclusion

Thank you for taking the time to read Vegetarian Keto Diet for Beginners: Lose Weight, Boost Brain Power and Increase Energy.

The aim of this book was to give you a good understanding of what the ketotarian diet is and where it originated from. We aimed to explain the principles that this diet has taken from both the ketogenic diet and other plant-based diets to provide you with a more wholesome, well-rounded, and healthy diet.

We also aimed to arm you with some techniques to get started on your ketotarian journey as well as some useful health tips that will take your life to the next level. We hope we have accomplished this, especially in the areas of weight loss, brain health, and energy levels. I hope you've learned a

Conclusion

lot of information that you can use to help improve your own life. I also hope you are more aware of the extent to which our diets dictate our health and how they can have an impact on the environment.

The next step is to get out there and start putting what you've learned into practice! Best of luck on your journey and don't forget to reward yourself along the way!

Finally, if you found this book useful in any way, a review on Amazon is always greatly appreciated! Thank you.

Ingram Content Group UK Ltd.
Milton Keynes UK
UKHW021320260623
424060UK00019B/437